M. Chay

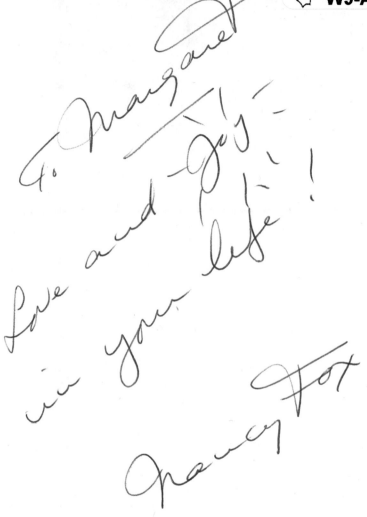

To Margaret

joy —

Love and

in your life!

Nancy Fox

How to Put
JOY
into Geriatric Care

How to Put
JOY
into Geriatric Care

by
Nancy Littell Fox

Illustrated by Patricia Collins
graduate of the
Pratt Institute of Art

ACKNOWLEDGMENTS

The author appreciates and thanks these publishers:

National Association for Practical Nurse Education and Service, Inc. (NAPNES), publishers of *Journal of Practical Nursing*, for permission to reprint in part or with adaptations the following five articles by Nancy Littell Fox: "Making Geriatric Nursing Creative," copyright © September, 1973 by NAPNES; "Rx: Range of Motion for the Funnybone," copyright © February, 1978 by NAPNES; "Aftermath of Stroke: Triumph or Tragedy?" copyright © April, 1975 by NAPNES; "To Make Meaningful Their Days," copyright © February, 1978 by NAPNES; and "A Good Birth, A Good Life—Why Not a Good Death?" copyright © October, 1974 by NAPNES.

The Rotarian for the poem "Eyes of the Beholder" by Lillian Doriah; copyright © December, 1974 by *The Rotarian*.

Harper & Brothers: *Masterpieces of Religious Verse*, edited by James Dalton Morrison, for two poems: "They Softly Walk," by Hugh Robert Orr, and "Victory in Defeat," by Edwin Markham; copyright © 1948 by Harper & Brothers.

For three limericks from Duell, Sloan and Pearce, *The Little Book of Limericks*, by H. I. Brock; copyright © 1947 by H. I. Brock.

Oxford University Press, N.Y.: *English Romantic Poetry and Prose*, edited by Russell Noyes, for "The Poison Tree" by William Blake. Copyright © 1965 by Oxford University Press.

Little, Brown & Company, Boston, Mass., for permission to use "Celery" and "The Parsnip" from *Verses From 1929* by Ogden Nash, copyright © 1941 by Ogden Nash.

Fourth Printing—1983

ISBN 0-9601874-1-3 Soft Cover
ISBN 0-9601874-2-1 Hard Cover

Library of Congress Catalog Card # 79-52166

Published by Geriatric Press, Inc.,
    1421 N.E. 8th Street, Bend Oregon 97701
Copyright 1979 by Nancy Littell Fox
Printed by St. Mary's Press, Winona, Minnesota
Illustrated by Patricia Collins

To "Mima," who said "YES" to Life;
who knew "How to Put Joy . . ."
and who, with enthusiasm,
remained ever alive
to the fragrance and fullness
of the world around her.

To All Who Provide Geriatric Care

May you "demonstrate that old age is not a defeat,
But a victory,
Not a punishment, but a privilege.
Let us hold ourselves responsive to their needs.
Let us be successful social innovators, and prove
That life, for the long-lived, can be
A many-splendored thing."*

*Ethel Percy Andrus, Ph.D., founder of American Association of Retired Persons and National Retired Teachers Association.

Contents

Preface

Rapidly sold out in the United States and Canada, the first editions of *How to Put JOY into Geriatric Care* confirmed the need for additional printings. Although the literature provides amply for the physical and psycho-social care of the elderly, the very idea of putting "JOY" into geriatrics, as stressed in this book, adds an important dimension for professionals and ancillary health care workers alike.

Widely used in nursing schools and for inservice training, the book opens the door to geriatric care—not as a ho-hum, depressing job to be done, but as a challenging career; one which allows for as many imaginative approaches as there are geriatric patients; one which can and should be, overall, a joyful, enriching experience.

Among the new topics introduced are:

> Gracious dining (How can this be achieved in an institutional setting?)
>
> Life-long learning (Can the mind, in old age, be kept alert?)
>
> Thoughts about the married couple in a nursing home
>
> Touch (What is that magic power of your hand?)
>
> Spiritual needs (Is nursing concerned with this aspect of total care?)

I dedicate this volume to my mother, "Mima," who demonstrated that life can be "a many-splendored thing."

Introduction

Zita Hall was an excellent geriatric unit. Proof of the pud-
ding was clearly evident in our records, often quoted by the
nursing staff: "Mrs. X has been a patient for ten years and
has never had a bedsore." "Mr. Y had a bedsore when he
came to us, but it has healed and he hasn't had any more in
his five years with us." You can't dispute facts like that: they
demonstrate good physical care.

The place was spotless and shining. The patients were
clean and neat. Too neat. Catheters flowed into plastic bags
on the side of the bed opposite the door, so as not to be of-
fensively visible. Nothing was out of place. But as administrator of the facility I felt that something was missing.

The problem had nothing to do with the physical care
nor with the plant itself. But the vacant expression on the
faces of the patients or the mute plea behind veiled eyes kept
haunting me. It was as if they were saying, "Hey, look at *me*."
And then I met Nancy Fox.

Nancy talked about "caring plans," not "nursing plans."
She talked about having aphasic patients give book reviews,
about stroke patients painting pictures; about staff-resident
sing-a-longs at the piano. "Nonsense," said the staff. But

Nancy kept hammering: "We must blend into the daily lives of *all* our residents," she said, "those activities which, till now, have been reserved for the lucky few who attend activity-room sessions."

Nancy planned individual birthday parties, Bible and poetry sharing, flower and pet shows. A double amputee was Queen of the Day when she won first prize for the Easter bonnet she had created. Gradually, the unit began to change. It wasn't always neat any more, but people were *alive*. They were persons again, with a thousand new interests and memories of old times to compare.

Morale among staff persons improved too. It didn't cost any money, just enthusiasm and a catalyst like Nancy to get the fire kindled. The activities were accepted slowly. It *did* take staff time to wheel everyone outside on a summer day for a lawn party. It meant staying with the patients rather than smoking another forbidden cigarette at the desk or sitting longer in the employees' lounge. But as the staff saw their charges come alive, they responded in the same way. Theirs was no longer just a job, maintaining crippled, ailing bodies; it was loving and caring for lovable people, each of whom had a lifetime of experience.

Nancy saved the biggest transition until the program was well established, then after consulting with the medical staff, she threw the bombshell. Remove the catheters and toilet train! The idea was carefully explained to participating patients and staff. Patients were eager; this meant regaining dignity. Staff was skeptical; it meant hard work. Somebody who had had a catheter for two years was offered *rehabilitation?* "Impossible" was the only comment. There were tears, accidents, frustration. But it worked, and it is harder to say who was prouder, staff or patients.

As an administrator I have to say that I witnessed a

radical change in our geriatrics unit once Mrs. Fox implemented some of her ideas. We were not only adding new years to their lives; we were adding new life to their years. In her book Mrs. Fox explains some of the ideas that she used as LPN floor supervisor, to transform a good geriatric unit into one where staff and patients were afforded the humanizing experience of beauty and love to grow in their humanity.

Sister Paschala Noonan
Director, St. Charles Jubilee Center
Brooklyn, New York

Sister Paschala Noonan, R.N., Sister of St. Dominic of St. Catherine, Kentucky, has had wide experience in the field of geriatric care. She has been a hospital administrator, a member of the American College of Hospital Administrators, and chairperson of the Nebraska State Board of Health. She has also served as assistant director of the Department of Pastoral Care in the Roman Catholic Diocese of Brooklyn, New York, serving over 120 nursing homes, and has served as a consultant on the national level on the country's responsibility to its elderly citizens.

Author's Note

"How depressing! How can you stand working with the aged?"

To one geriatric nurse, this question comes as no surprise, but to another?

"*Stand* it?" she answers. "I enjoy it. What a challenge—this reaching out for the highest potential in each one of our old persons! My life has been greatly enriched."

"But to tell the truth, isn't it depressing in those nursing homes?"

"Only when the staff allows its."

"*Allows* it?"

Yes, it is true—much depends upon you, the staff. We discovered this at our Hillside Home, where today gloom is no longer taken for granted. There was a time when the oppressive atmosphere hovering over the place like a heavy fog, took its toll in staff-patient morale; in recurring illness (psychosomatic and otherwise); and in staff turnover, that endless hiring-firing-quitting marathon so crippling to the average nursing home. And the resident, bewildered by this whirling kaleidoscope of strange, unhappy faces, was the biggest loser. Besides, the nurse and her assistant who worked begrudgingly seemed to spend three times as much energy as the one taking a "hurray, another workday" approach.

It was the routine at Hillside, the deadly, monotonous, unrelieved routine that had kept staff and residents depressed, dulled our senses, and clipped our wings. I became convinced of this one clear, moonless night as I glanced out the window while I raced down the hall. There in the sky were myriads of stars fairly blazing with energy, a beautiful sight. I stopped a moment, to marvel, and as I did, my thoughts fell on old Mr. Crowell in Room 79. There he lay, sound asleep, lights out as always by 8 p.m. I recalled how more than once he had tried to share with us his fascination with, and knowledge of, the stars, but our response had always been merely, "How nice!"

The following night, instead of pajamas, we handed Mr. Crowell his jacket, wheeled him outdoors and, for a magic fifteen minutes, watched his midsummer night's dream come true. Enthralled once again by the mysteries of the universe, "This is really living!" he cried.

Really living? The words haunted us. Isn't this what Hillside should be all about? He, and all the residents, *let them be alive!* On a lovely day, why should those outdoor chairs be unoccupied? What if more flowerbeds and shrubs were to be planted? Why not a birdbath? Goldfish pond? Why not some community club to launch a fund-raising project for this? Surely these simple pleasures mean more to the elderly than to others, for, with a lessened spring in the step, they have the time now for enjoyment.

We had been slaves to routine. We had not recognized patients as people; had not added lustre to their lives, nor provided enough outlets for creative self-expression. Therapists and activities directors couldn't possibly reach every resident—they worked with only a few, and for only a small part of each month. There had to be a grand reversal of our whole way of life, beginning with *us,* with the determination to reach our own highest potential; to expand our spirits, imagination, and initiative; to become more alive to the fragrance and fullness of the world about us. To the extent that we did this for ourselves, to that degree our own *joie de vivre* would rub off on the lives of our residents. The joy in them was there — had always been there. It was simply waiting to be tapped. And how we tapped it — that is what this book is all about — all the ways I've seen it work, not only at Hillside, but in other homes where good things are happening. Everything in this book is real, it is firsthand experience, drawn from years of observation and employment in nursing homes across the land. (Names have been changed, of course.) It was written to share with you our enthusiasm as we look around now and find each of our residents living just a little more fully. And loving it.

In the process of reversing our way of life at Hillside, we made an important discovery, and that is that joy exists on many levels. On one level, we see it in Mrs. Baker's eyes, as she puts the final stitch on her afghan, or in Mr. Putman's expression when, after months, he takes his first step. But there is a deeper level of joy which comes from the sharing of ourselves, not only with the living, active residents, but with the dying. And so, in our last chapter, as we move into a private-home setting (where some of you, at times, are asked to "special" a patient), we share the actual joy of a terminal patient in her experience of a peaceful death. For Augusta, and for all those of deep religious faith, the passing from this world may mean the coming "into God's presence in the fullness of joy."

Someone said: "Let love be the music that we play." How natural, then, how simple, with love as our background music, to put joy into geriatric care! And so, my nurse colleagues, don't hold back. The sky is your limit — that very same star-studded sky Mr. Crowell wants to tell you about.

Our continuing hope for Hillside? That each precious person here, in this home away from home, may have life, and have it more abundantly.

N. L. F.

*Not all the staff, especially students or first-year nurses and nursing
assistants, have had the chance to see the dramatic things which can
and do happen in the good nursing home. Let's watch, now, as a creative staff revolutionizes the drab lives of Mrs. Stevens and "Tillie, the
Tyrant." This is the great joy of*

1 Making Geriatric Nursing Creative

In her nineties, Mrs. Stevens had not spoken a word in years.
She sat alone most of the day, her head bent nearly to her
lap. Everything had been done for, not with, her. All her
sense of personal worth had long since slipped down the
drain.

"Our goal for Mrs. Stevens," resolved the Hillside staff,
"is to keep trying till we get through to her." And so, day
after day, we probed her mind, searching for the key—the
one memory that would bring back a sparkle to her eyes.
Finally, the jackpot question:

"Mrs. Stevens, do you like flowers?"

A sudden change of expression came over her lovely face.

"Mrs. Stevens," repeated the nurse, "what kinds of flowers did you grow in your garden?"

Raising her eyes for the first time, she started naming flowers, one after another—dahlias, roses, tulips, until, breathlessly and excitedly, she had named no less than ten varieties. The delighted nurse hugged Mrs. Stevens, said, "I'll be right back!" and rushed to tell the rest of the staff what had happened.

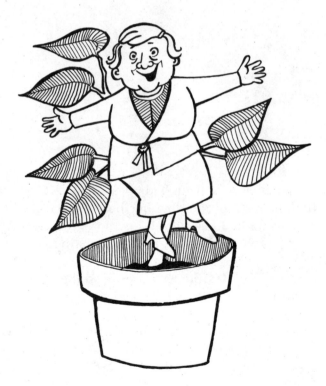

Mrs. Stevens' interest in flowers was our cue. We provided flower pots and helped her do her own planting. We deluged her with flower picture books. We talked flowers with her during meals, during manicures, tubbings—any old time. She unfolded and blossomed out like one of her rosebuds!

Gradually, Mrs. Stevens lost her shyness and joined in group activities. She knew that we cared. The crowning joy was the day she consented to sing before the entire group. With head high, she walked to the center of the room and opened up loud and clear with her favorite: "Daisy, Daisy, Give Me Your Answer, Do," with confidence that reflected her newfound inner happiness. There was not one dry eye in the room. We knew that for Mrs. Stevens, life was once again worth living.

In trying out this new approach to our residents, we thought of a feisty old lady whom we had nicknamed "Tillie, the Tyrant." Wasn't there some way we could reach her? I was elected to try. This was a real challenge. Tillie delighted in kicking anyone in the shins who came within reach— socked you right in the face whenever she took a notion. Cussed you in language that would make a longshoreman blush. Hadn't left her chair in two years. That was old Tillie Finnegan. You'd best keep out of her way, or so we believed.

A bad temper and can't walk? Intending to check out those two assumptions, I ventured to her a pleasant "Hello!" I was standing too close.

"Don't you 'hello' *me*, you rotten old blankety-blank," she retorted, swinging her fist and simultaneously landing a hefty kick just below my knee.

Wincing, but determined to keep cool, I answered, "Tillie Finnegan—why, you must be Irish! I just love that Irish spirit! My, how those sparkling blue eyes dance when you flash your hash like that! What spirit! What spunk! It's got to be the Irish in you?"

Narrowing her eyes in utter disbelief at my reaction, she composed herself, admitted to being Irish, and proudly proceeded to brag about her parents from Dublin.

Before long, Tillie began to thaw. A marked change showed in the old battle-ax. Her temper diminished. She allowed me to give her walking lessons and in two months was stomping down the hall, with a pleasant greeting for all.

Soon this newfound freedom brought on some new deviltry. She began sneaking downstairs to the men's dormitory, and even into their bathrooms. They called her "Mrs. Pest." But she respected my stern admonitions that ladies were not welcomed there and didn't even take a swing at me. Before long, Tillie became the darling of the entire home. Everyone adored her flashing eyes and wit, which now she was able to channel into constructive activities as she widened her enthusiasm for other people.

When we see how changes can be made in the very different (but equally difficult) cases of a Mrs. Stevens and a Tillie in a nursing home, is it any wonder that I am challenged by the question "Is it depressing?" It need not be depressing. Working with the aged can be fulfilling, with rewards that stretch into infinity. What a challenge for the nurse—this reaching for the highest potential in each of those dear old persons; a chance to help them live "the greatest number of good hours." And in turn, what they give to us! The enrichment of our own lives is incalculable.

Joy in geriatric care?
Then why not

2 Rx: Range-of-Motion—
for the Funny Bone?

Doctor orders R.O.M. for the femur, the fibula—for every bone except one. He forgets the funny bone. And yet, if immobilized, it, too, will atrophy. Even we nurses know that when a new resident comes to Hillside, he brings more than just a suitcase. He may already have a well-developed funny bone.

What's this—a nurse *prescribing?* Certainly. Humor therapy. Isn't laughter the best medicine? It may not come in bottles but oh, how humor can heal! A sure-fire remedy for stress—a remedy often needed, as well, by the nurse—by me, for example, on the day I entered the cubicle shared by Waldo and Jasper.*

*We never use patients' first names except with their permission. Some like it, others feel strongly that a more formal relationship with the staff is preferable. This we always try to respect.

Waldo, I must explain, was the victim of an old eye injury and proud possessor of a removable glass eye. At that moment he was reading the paper, his back to Jasper. And Jasper, despite the "no-smoking" sign, was smoking in bed.

"O.K. for you!" I snorted, "hand them over, Jasper."

"But Nurse," he wailed, "Doc says I can smoke if Waldo watches me."

"Waldo is *not* watching you," I replied firmly.

"Beg your pardon, Ma'am, but he *is* watching me."

By now I was livid. But when I glanced towards Waldo's back, I let out a whoop that you could hear down the hall. For there was Waldo, still reading, but over his left shoulder, gripped between his left thumb and forefinger, was peering the glass eye.

It was "watching" all right—it was "looking" straight at Jasper!

And so, why not put "humor" on your med tray? Administer Q.D. to every resident. For who can stay hurt while emitting a hearty laugh?

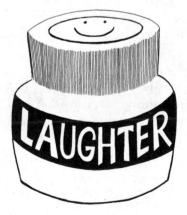

Talk about therapeutic! When your patient laughs, why does he (she) feel so good? Because pure, delicious oxygen pours in—penetrates every last pulmonary alveolus. And because laughter, like a warm tropical sun, soothes away tension. Why not range-of-motion, then, for that all-too-often-ignored os humerus?

Not that we toss cheer bouquets glibly, as one scatters seed to the birds. Residents are smart—they read between the smiles—may even feel that they're getting the brush-off. No, but along with your TLC, try something new. The light touch. The trick is to know each resident and watch your timing. Phenomenal, how it forestalls a crisis, as happened the day one of our Hillside nurses prescribed laughter for Mrs. Bates. (And the bonus? Nurse Peg spared this person what could have been a shattering loss of self-esteem.)

Her morale at rock bottom, Mrs. Bates just "knew" that her aphasia was incurable. As she sat there, frustrated, in walked Peg with the dinner tray, setting it down before her. In response, with a hefty shove, the patient sent the whole thing crashing—gravy, soup, pie—a splattered mess all over the new carpet.

Now you or I might have gnashed our teeth and pounced on the lady with a pompous sermon. But not Peg. She understood that Mrs. Bates needed no additional pile-up of remorse. For a moment Peg paused—then, calmly: "Mrs. Bates, for your information, I've been studying the carpet manufacturer's instructions on 'Proper Care for Nursing Home Carpets.' He recommends: 'To insure long wear and brilliant lustre, douse carpet frequently and thoroughly with gravy, pea soup, raspberry jello, etc.'"

Mrs. Bates gasped. The knotted nerves loosened. She began to titter. It seemed she would burst as her laughter became uproarious. Her wheelchair rattled, almost collapsed. Peg put her arm around her, and together they enjoyed the absurdity.

As a geriatric nurse, what are *your* aggravations? Are you on top? Who gives you the most "trouble"? Why? Ever try the light touch?

Humor therapy, however, need not be entirely up to the nurse. As we suspect, most patients come in with an already activated funny bone. Often it is they, themselves, through humor, who alleviate their own tensions. This we can encourage. I remember old Mr. Grady, awakened at dawn when I dropped a pitcher of water. At first hopping mad, judging from his unquotable language, he regained his composure and quipped: "Where else could I get ice water at five in the morning!"

Or, like the newly admitted blind woman, who was jabbed in the cheek when a busy nurse hastily offered a spoonful of spinach. "What's this?" she cried, and was told that because she was blind, she had to be fed. "Fiddle," snapped she. "I can feed myself. After all, *I* know where my mouth is!" and proceeded to demonstrate.

Fun, laughter, humor. Picture the nursing home where staff and residents look at the light side, where callers exclaim: "My, how I love to visit this place—it's so *cheerful*!" Or where the residents tell you: "Of course! We don't stop laughing when we get old. We get old when we stop laughing!"

And so, Nurse, start looking for all the funny bones you can find. They're still functioning, so bring them to light. And if it's humor we prescribe for the well-being of our patients—come on, let's get going with that R.O.M. That's it— abduction, adduction, extension—flex that funny bone.

To function or to fossilize—*is* there a question? Show those residents, as Peg did, and, in turn, they'll show *you*, that

> No matter how grouchy you're feeling,
> Your smile is more or less healing.
> It grows like a wreath
> All around your front teeth,
> Thus preserving your face from congealing!

For joyous geriatrics,
what about

3 A Kitten in a Care Plan

That title—it's got to be a mistake!

But no, it isn't a mistake. There *should* be a kitten in a care plan. *And* a puppy. And a cat. And a dog.

Unheard of? Alas, yes, in most nursing homes. Absurd? *Not* at all. Hear this:

Twice a month a Colorado humane society drives its "Pet-Mobile" to four area nursing homes. Yes, and how the excited residents reach out for a pet to love and, for an hour, to go mad with the joy of snuggling it close!

As old Mrs. Billings presses "Whitey" to her bosom, it's puppy-love from the start. And Mr. Rodrigues, lame and lonesome, gently strokes "Mitten"—that likewise lonesome, but oh-so-cuddly kitten with the one black paw.

Well now, wouldn't you call this "Therapy" with a capital T? It's positively electric, the way it turns on the residents, lights them up, jolts them out of lethargy. Suddenly they're like kids at the circus, for many relate better to a friendly, furry animal than to—pardon the comparison—a doctor or nurse.

But if pet therapy in geriatric care is so successful, why has this need been ignored? Why is the Pet-Mobile a rarity instead of a familiar sight? Because pets carry germs? True, they do, as does the staff which daily enters the nursing home. Or is it because pets may soil? True, they may, nature being what it is. But in five years of this Colorado project, it has rarely happened. And if it does? Well, the world won't stall on its axis.

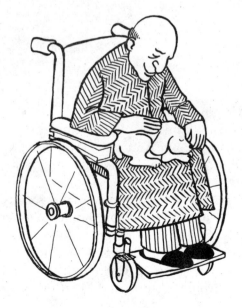

Pet therapy? You're still skeptical? Then consider:

1) There's special rapport between animals and old people. They respond to one another's feelings of helplessness.
2) Pets speak the language of the deaf, the blind, the confused, the physically impaired.
3) Animals are uncritical. (Ever see a kitten object to arthritis?) They cozy up to anyone who loves them.
4) Although all people need some kind of physical contact, it is these, the institutionalized, who rarely, if ever, get enough.

Bouquets to Mr. Phil Arkow of the Pikes Peak Region Humane Society for providing this imaginative service and to the nursing home administrators who appreciate its value. "We're more than just an animal pound," says Mr. Arkow, "we're a community resource."

Quick, look out the window! Today's the day. Here comes that Pet-Mobile. Ready, pets and patients, for a grand reunion? And Nurse, for the residents, today it will be *cats*, not Chlorpromazine; *dogs*, not Diazepam. And this "pet-therapy" thing—isn't that just a fancy name for heavy doses of undiluted love?

Just watch those residents—their joy, their shining eyes! A lump comes to your throat—the way they adore that bark, that miaow at one end, that wag on the other, and all that love in between—they gather it in, cherishing every moment. For is not this the world's most appreciative group, the institutionalized aged?

If a pet in hand is worth ten in the pound, then why not? Is there a pup for your patients? A kitten in a care plan? Not just *a* care plan, Nurse.

Your care plan?

To spark their spirits,
which shall it be—

4 Pub—or Public Opinion?

Nurse Kathy and I are on our coffee break. It appears that I have caught her off guard.

"A pub? In a nursing home? Wine? Beer? *Here*—at Sunhaven? Nancy, you're nuts!"

My friend is aghast. "Why, this town would send a posse to picket the place. Don't you know we'd lose all financial backing?"

"But wait, Kathy. Don't *you* know we'd be right in the camp of Hippocrates himself? Why, even two thousand years ago *he* knew the therapeutic powers of wine! And what about all those professional journals—so much written lately about doctors and psychologists recommending it. There are lots of scientific studies showing how wine reduces tension, and really now, Kathy, isn't there enough tension around here? Think how it could improve staff-patient rapport. Heaven knows, and so do you, how here at Sunhaven we overshoot our quota of aggravations!"

"Well anyway," replied Kathy, "I must say we're not exactly famous for innovative ideas. Sometimes I really do believe that Sunhaven operates on the premise that change—*any* change in routine—is either un-American or un-Christian. Maybe something *should* be done to reverse that stuffy image."

"Got to get back to work," I said, draining my cup to the dregs. "But can't you just picture a predinner social hour, say twice a week, with a little glass of wine to spark their spirits—"

"Served in a special pub room with a cozy atmosphere—" interrupted Kathy, herself suddenly getting the picture. "Imagine, a glass of sparkling wine—what a stimulant to appetites, not to mention conversation! As it is now, they're all in such a rut."

I sat back down again. The subject intrigues us both. Kathy bet her class pin that Dr. Roth, and maybe Dr. Brown, would go along with the idea that a little nightcap for some patients might eliminate the need for "sleepers"—those bromides and barbituates that can cause mental confusion. "Say, Kathy," I exclaimed, "that rut they're all in, isn't that the *best* reason of all to try something new? Too many of them are suffering from the 'blahs.' "

At that we both jumped up. "Great Scott, look at the time!"

That night, as I lie in bed, my imagination takes wings. I see our old people preparing for the weekly "Candlelight

Sherry Hour"—the ladies donning their prettiest dresses, the men their sharpest ties. Necklaces, nailpolish—and there's old Mrs. Foggarty, grinning as she dabs on her rouge:

> I haven't lost the bloom of youth,
> My eyes still have a twinkle,
> My face is smooth, but here and there
> My mirror has a wrinkle!

And now, still dreaming, I see the residents gathered together, each with a little stemmed glass. Someone is pouring a light *vin rosé*. The record-player is twirling a Victor Herbert waltz; all who can are engaged in spirited chatter. Someone else is pouring fruit-juice for those who cannot, may not, or prefer not to take wine, and they, too, are wearing happy faces to replace the old overhanging gloomy expressions. Tension, tempers, all have faded away.

Wine therapy at Sunhaven? No, in my dream, Kathy and I aren't "nuts." We think it's a gem of an idea! Who knows, it might end up with a bit of dancing!

By now, thrashing around in bed and on the verge of awakening, I hear a voice—I can't tell whose—saying: "It would be too costly; I'm not sure they'd enjoy it; *we really must consider public opinion.*"

I wake up with a start.

Earlier, we mentioned "scientific studies." What has been found, you'd like to know. How does wine therapy actually meet the needs of many elderly residents? Results of one such study,* documented by Alice Fitzgerald, R.N.,

---

*Alice Fitzgerald, R.N., "Pilot Project Using Wine Therapy with Long-Term Patients," *Journal of Gerontological Nursing*, October, 1975.

were summarized after two months, then again after fifteen. Each participant was observed as to effects (benefits, or lack of them), and as to any changes in physical or mental status. The final consensus of residents, staff, and families: "The program should be continued."

After the first two months, there was marked improvement in living habits of most of the twenty-three participants; an attitude of more awareness for their peers, staff, and general environment. When the wine was served in two installments of two-and-a-half ounces each, with a ten-to-

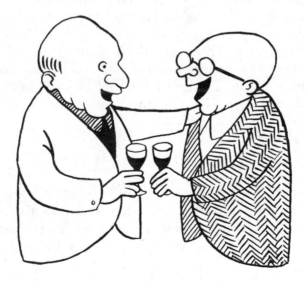

PUB—or . . .

fifteen-minute interval, socialization occurred at a more leisurely pace. Snacks were available, and often there was planned activity to enhance the pleasure.

After fifteen months, assessments showed that for some, nutritional habits had improved. There were fewer complaints, better socialization, and more participation in activities. All stated they slept well, none using "sleepers."

The next day, Kathy and I are back together, having coffee. Here at Sunhaven, which shall it be, we wonder—

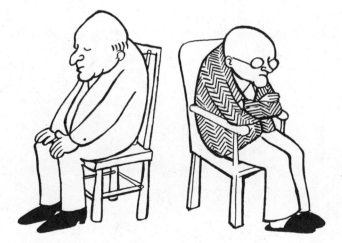

PUBLIC OPINION?

5 There's Lots of Music Left in an Old Fiddle!

Music hath more than just charms. It hath potential for joyous geriatric rejuvenation.

"What's going on around here?" grumped our Hillside administrator on the phone. "Even with my office door shut, I can hear the racket!"

"Seeing is believing," replied the nurse. "Go look in the lounge."

As the administrator marched down the hall, the din increased. At the door, he stopped short. Then blinked. No, he couldn't believe it. First he caught sight of me at the piano. That in itself set him off laughing. I'm no Van Cliburn, but caring not a hoot, I was hacking away at "Happy Days Are Here Again," while there they were—the whole geriatric gang—in a cozy circle singing, clapping, stamping their feet. Not even a Times Square New Year's shindig could match the spirit, the shine, in all those old eyes!

But this was only the beginning. The next day, reassembled, the residents begged for hymns, like "Work for the Night Is Coming"—I hadn't heard it in years—and hoped that the Man Upstairs didn't mind their rhythm-clapping to *that*. The third day it was patriotic favorites, sung with such gusto ("Glory Halleluiah") that the walls nearly came unglued. And so each day thereafter the singing went on, always beginning with "Hail, hail the gang's all here!" until the songfest was a daily ritual. And for the first time in the institution's history, the residents were united in a common, joyous bond.

Let it be known, though, that before this phenomenon came to pass, the atmosphere around here had been pretty —shall we say "morose"? Downright depressing. No interaction. Take old Mrs. Peabody, that "proper Bostonian"—

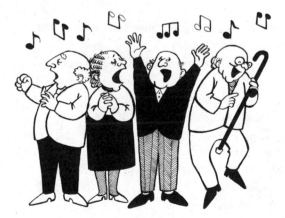

she wouldn't communicate. "They have no culture!" she'd complain. Or old Mr. Gonzales with his thick accent. "One of those illegal aliens," some of the others suspected. Or that feisty old Mrs. Grady. "Nobody understands me," she'd fuss. "They're ignorant about Ireland—don't know it's the only spot on earth God really likes." And skinny Miss Sims— aphasic, but that evil temper, why you'd think she was the Queen of Sheba, the way she'd wave her arms and try to boss the staff! Not to mention timid, peaked little Mr. Chiswick over there, afraid of his own shadow. And all those others, so lost in their own woes.

But look at them now. Not even a ghost could scare them away from their daily music hour. It's positively magic! And oh, the smiles, the laughter, patting, hugging that goes on! (I tell you, if the nations would sing together, all wars would cease!)

Music. That's all it took. And now, not only friends and families, including the kiddies, drop by, but even the administrator sometimes joins in to harmonize with his big bass voice. Which reminds me—would you like to hear a well-whispered secret around here? You know, for *years* that man has advertised this home in his brochure as "one big happy family." But that must have been with tongue in cheek. Now he's safe. For, with a new spirit of joy, of warmth, of closer ties among the residents, that is exactly what it is—one big happy family.

As we said before, this singing was just a starter. We soon discovered other hidden charms that music hath—things we should have known about long ago from people like Ruth Bright,* who has been plugging music therapy for years—

*Music therapist, New South Wales Health Department, Australia. See her book, *Music in Geriatric Care*, published in 1973 by St. Martin's Press, Inc., 175 5th Ave., New York, N.Y. 10010.

not only singing, but using instruments such as castanets, drums, cymbals, and handbells. In the hope, now, that a word to the wise is sufficient (wise nursing staffs, that is), let me quote from the flap of her book:

> . . . she sees music as providing an emotive quality often lacking in medical treatment, whether physical or psychological, which give each individual a chance to express himself as a person, not simply as a patient.
>
> By providing the opportunity for shared interest and activity, music can assist in the socialization of the elderly . . . The associative powers of music can build a happy atmosphere in group work and help to overcome the feelings of confusion, loss and inadequacy so unfortunately common among the elderly. Musical activity is useful in improving motivation and reinforcing the learning of exercises in physical therapy involving the relearning of motor skills or the learning of new skills to compensate for loss or impairment.

Music hath charms, all right. It hath potential, as we've seen, for joyful, geriatric rejuvenation. With residents participating, it belongs in every nursing home in the land.

Well, perhaps our little geriatric singing gang may not be asked to premiere at the Metropolitan, nor to set forth on a nationwide concert tour. But they'll keep that "music in the air," for there's one thing they know for sure, the old proverb:

> When we sigh, nobody hears us;
> When we sing, *everybody* hears us.

*One of the charms
that music hath is—
more music.*

6 "May I Have the Next Dance?"

Something unforgettable happened one afternoon at Hillside. Most of the visitors had gone, and a group of residents remained in the lounge, waiting for supper to be served. Whether it was because this was Saturday and Nurse McClain was in a festive mood, or whether she was inspired by the recent sing-along, we can't say, but suddenly, stepping over to the long-dormant record-player, she put on an old record. As the compelling rhythm of the "Missouri Waltz" broke the silence, she stood back to observe reactions.

At once mouths began to curl upwards. Several residents started to hum along with the tune. Legs and arms twitched

43

to the rhythm. But then, suddenly, at the Hillside Home, history was made—for out of his cubicle doorway emerged Mr. Vessini, all 92 years of him. (Thirty-five witnesses will attest to his age.) Clapping his hands and calling out "Wahoo," he grabbed Nurse McClain and propelled her toward the center of the room.

Miss McClain was speechless. What if he had a heart attack right here before everyone? What if the supervisor should appear? But how could she now back off, how could she reject a man with a shine in his eyes she never before had noticed? Mr. Vessini was inspired. He gripped her shoulder, took her hand, and moving with long, light steps, caught her up irresistibly in the spirit of the moment.

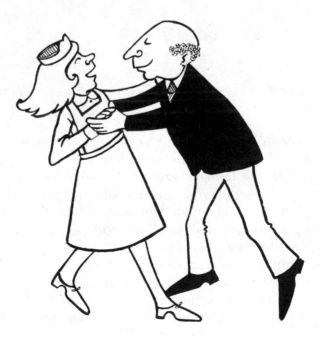

The group of spectators was delighted. Soon, another couple joined in. Then another. Then, two women, noting the shortage of gentlemen, stood up, locked arms, and together tripped the "light fantastic." In fact, the *whole scene* was fantastic!

For a few fleeting moments, all hunger pangs dissolved into thin air as a happy electricity filled the room.

Within one month, a new record collection was acquired for the Hillside lounge. And Saturday nights became the "dance-and-date" night for the ambulatory residents. Many emerged from their cocoons to join the frolic.

Hillside is obviously a special place. Particularly when an old charmer like Mr. Vessini can grab you and say: "May I have the next dance?"

And now,
to open up joyous vistas—
to help them spread their wings—

7 Let There Be Poetry

"Well," I shrugged, "it gives them something to pass the time!"

Thinking back to that remark I flung out about the poetry group, I shudder. Such ignorance! For now I know that at Hillside, or in any good nursing home, poetry therapy is as important as physical, or other, therapy. It has been called the "scientific application of literature towards a therapeutic goal."

Poetry, like music, stimulates the emotions, the intellect. It has a way of drawing a person out, helps him (her) to articulate his feelings, orients him to reality. Not every geriatric

47

patient benefits, but anyone can gather a group together to try it—to let who will, enjoy a poem and share reactions.

An expert in this field, Dr. Arthur Lerner* tells of Tom, a frustrated resident who read a poem that he felt really helped him. It was William Blake's "The Poison Tree."

> I was angry with my friend:
> I told my wrath, my wrath did end.
> I was angry with my foe:
> I told it not, my wrath did grow.

Tom told his group that he had never displayed his feelings and that the poem helped him deal with this problem.

For some of us, poetry seems remote—something kept back in our past. But do you remember how, when you were a child, a poem brought sighs, smiles, or tears? And how, in your mind's eye, you could "see" the "host of golden daffodils, fluttering and dancing in the breeze"? Who can forget the bubbling excitement of "'Twas the Night Before Christmas"? Remember how weepy you were when, after Little Boy Blue died, there, so forlornly, sat the little toy dog and toy soldier, covered with dust, waiting in vain for their little master?

Poetry, by "catching" our thoughts, puts us in touch with our selves. We reach into the subconscious, or soar to the far away, or into our here-and-now feelings. The therapist uses it to unearth and soothe our rough spots of guilt, hos-

*Dr. Lerner is professor of psychology at Los Angeles City College, California, and director of poetry therapy at Woodview-Calabasas Hospital, Calabasas, California. In addition to being a widely published poet, he is also founder and director of the Poetry Therapy Institute, Encino, California.

tility, or hopelessness. And again, like music, it can calm the restless mind.

Even without a professional therapist, any nursing home can organize an informal group for poetry readings. At Hillside, it began with a visitor, Mrs. Cades, herself a published poet, who inspired interest among eleven residents. With permission for a weekly session, she provided suitable poems, reading them with feeling and encouraging listeners to participate in readings and discussion. From this spark we opened the Hillside doors for this new and wonderful outlet. You, too, may have someone in your community, a warm person, known for his or her love of poetry. Ask her to share her love with your ready audience. The experience will be a rich one for her as well as for the group. We found that the poetry group also had another function, in that it was one more good way to strengthen the ties between the nursing home and the community.

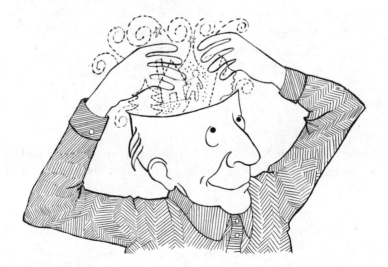

For the older person, the sharing of concerns through poetry is especially important because when bottled up, he feels misunderstood, or easily falls prey to despair. As happened to Mrs. Greer.

Since her daughter's death, Mrs. Greer had been inconsolable. None of our attempts to reach out to her had lightened the burden. In mentioning this to Mrs. Cades, I unexpectedly paved the way for something good. Mrs. Cades understood. Visiting Mrs. Greer privately in her room, she asked her simply to listen quietly to a poem. This is what she read:

They Softly Walk
They are not dead who live
In hearts they leave behind.
In those whom they have blessed
They live a life again,
And shall live through the years
Eternal life, and grow
Each day more beautiful
As time declares their good,
Forgets the rest, and proves
Their immortality.

Hugh Robert Orr

After a moment's silence, Mrs. Greer asked her to read it again, then to copy it out for her. Parts of it she memorized. Before long, she seemed better able to adjust to her loss.

And here's one that struck a chord for Mr. Hansen, who, widowed early in life, felt he had suffered more than his share:

Victory in Defeat
Defeat may serve as well as victory
To shake the soul and let the glory out.
When the great oak is straining in the wind,
The boughs drink in new beauty, and the trunk
Sends down a deeper root on the windward side.
Only the soul that knows the mighty grief
Can know the mighty rapture. Sorrows come
To stretch our spaces in the heart for joy.

Edwin Markham

All of the group responded to another one that described the tough road of life—the steep ascent, taken by the brave, not by weaklings who walk the rose-strewn path. Each seemed to feel, "That's the story of my life!"

And finally, without discussing specific poems of patriotism, of a spiritual nature, of parenthood, of the beauty of nature—for there are poems on every topic of concern to man—we will just mention the joys of humorous poetry. Nearly all patients adore the silly, funny, ridiculous ones. And I nominate for Poet Laureate of Nursing Homes none other than Ogden Nash, whose Golden Trashery of Ogden Nashery has tickled many a geriatric rib at these poetry sessions, especially the little miniverses such as:

The parsnip, children,   *or*   Celery raw
   I repeat   Develops the jaw
Is simply an anemic beet   But celery stewed
Some people call the pars-   Is more quietly chewed!
   nip edible
Myself, I call the claim in-
   credible!

Older people also enjoy limericks, which sometimes

help them to laugh at themselves. Like this one, for example:

> These places abound in the old
> Who do nothing but quibble and scold,
> Discussing their tumors
> And stock-market rumors,
> They are tangibly covered with mold!
>
> *George Libaire*

How relaxed the atmosphere—what joy to hear the hoots of merriment when they catch the spirit of nonsense in such as:

> There was a young lady of Byde
> Who ate a green apple and died;
> The apple fermented
> Inside the lamented,
> And made cider inside her inside.

followed by:

> There was a young man from Peru
> Who found a large mouse in his stew.
> Said the waiter, "Don't shout,
> And wave it about,
> Or the rest will be wanting one too!"

Poetry in the nursing home—just a pastime? How *could* I have said such a thing! No, no, a thousand times no. It is infinitely more, especially when the leader is someone to whom the patients can relate. How, then, are we to help our patients spread their wings? How may we put more life, more joy, into geriatric care?

Poetry.

That's how!

That joyous little plus—
It's called: "Gracious Dining."
(Ask Mrs. Wade.)

8 Dinner Is Served!

The year is 1966. It is sundown as a crack locomotive, the "20th Century Limited" speeds its way from Chicago to New York. Suddenly the travelers are startled by the sound of a brass gong.

"Dinner is served!" announces the headwaiter as he goes from car to car spreading the glad news. Passengers perk up. Many are formally attired for tonight's dinner will be a special event. Through the corridors they thread their way to the dining car, once considered the "last word" in elegance, with its red velvet drapes and carved woodwork— reminders of a by-gone era.

The ladies are seated, a carnation corsage pinned on each shoulder. Irish linen cloths and bowls of fresh red roses adorn every table. And now, impeccably dressed, smiling waiters set before us steaming platters of delectable baked "Duck a l'Orange"—as dramatic as a Buckingham Palace dinner party. And we feel like royalty, too, as our glasses are filled, "on the house," with a delicate Rhine wine. Very quickly, strangers become friends as they strike up animated conversations from table to table.

Beneath the surface, however, an air of sadness prevails—nostalgia you could call it. For tonight's gala dinner will soon become history—the last to be served in this setting. The magnificent 20th Century Limited is making its final run.

I glance out the window. The sun is just setting as my thoughts soar back to my hometown, and to the beautiful health-care center where I work. A simple idea strikes me— how ideal it would be if such facilities could even approach this concept of gracious dining! And yet, at our Juniper Health Home, despite its limitations, the "Dinner-Is-Served" department deserves a blue ribbon. For there, too, each resident is made to feel he or she is somebody special. And for this, we can thank the indomitable Mrs. Wade, Food Services Supervisor, who has presided over the meals, it seems, since the Year One.

At the Juniper Home, the goal of the nutrition program goes far beyond the mere balancing of nutrients. "Meals are meant," says Mrs. Wade, "for taste, nostril and eye-appeal; to keep our residents joyous and alert; to be the highlight of their day."

"Would you like white bread or brown, dear?" she asks, or "Would you prefer your juice now or later, Mr. Sills?" She wants to allow for personal decision-making because it is Mrs. Wade's unswerving conviction that when individuality gives way to mass treatment, dignity is sacrificed. Here, no such sacrifice is imminent, we feel, as long as Mrs. Wade reigns as "Queen-of-the-Cuisine."

Let me describe a meal at the Juniper Home. Take an imaginary peek at the dinner served the day before I boarded this train for my vacation. By the manner in which it was prepared and served, it conveyed an unmistakable message to each resident—just as clearly as the backrub does—"We care about you. We care about your tastes, your feelings, about you, as a person." The meal symbolized the quality of care to which this home is committed. Aware that taste and appetite of older people may be less acute, you notice the portions are small. A subtle way of saying: "Have some more!"

Every dish (and Mrs. Wade inspects each one) must be a work of art in variety, texture and color. Look at that attractive appetizer, the half grapefruit—scalloped around the rim and with a maraschino cherry in the center! Or that sprig of parsley decorating the meat! And those hot rolls served from a pretty basket and later those pink and green after-dinner mints. These are all little creative touches re-

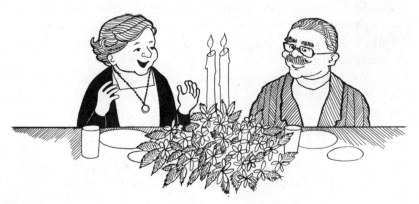

quiring only moments of time plus imagination to enhance the delights of dining.

Royal treatment, too, is accorded those on special diets. At their table, do you notice the little unsweetened or unsalted goodies—relishes or snacks—to tempt the palate? "Well, Mr. Larsen, are you enjoying your dinner?" asks Mrs. Wade as, like a mother hen, she hovers lovingly over a resident. (Mrs. Wade knows each resident by name and loves them all.)

"Bare tables? Here at Juniper? Perish the thought!" she says, pointing to the colorful, bright cloths which, although necessarily of plastic, look like real linen. And those fresh flowers brought in by staff members from churches, or from their own gardens. And during dinner, soft background music eases tension, relaxes tired bodies. Nobody hurries, the staff moves about quietly. And never, ever, will you encounter what Mrs. Wade considers to be the cardinal culinary crime: the clattering of dishes from the kitchen area.

Yes, a dinner at the Juniper Home means good food, smiles and leisurely enjoyment. And if, because of her workload and that of the dietary staff, the meals cannot quite be classified as gourmet, more importantly, they are served with pride and care, just as they are tonight, on this train. And so, Mrs. Wade, long may you live until you, too, make your final run!

Although I'll not be traveling this route again, I'll never forget this festive dinner. It makes me more aware than ever of Mrs. Wade's old-fashioned devotion to gracious dining. And I can't help but smile—no, marvel—at the shine in the eyes of our residents when mealtime approaches. No wonder they perk up, as we did tonight on the 20th Century Limited, at the sound of those magic words: "Dinner Is Served!"

Life-Long Learning?
One of the joys of geriatrics is our effort . . .

9 "To Keep Open the Paths"

"Now what's that smiling eighty-three-year-old doing up there in the cockpit of a plane?"

"Why that's Mrs. Evelyn Hobday. She's taking flying lessons!"

"And why is that ninety-year-old man signing what looks like a contract?"

"Why that's *just* what it is! He's signing a new teaching contract for the coming year."

"But what's that sharp-eyed old woman doing filling a syringe?"

"Why that's Dr. Maile Kachel, still practicing medicine at the age of ninety-four."

Friends, we fool you not! These are bona fide examples of mental competence in later life. Not surprising, really, for researchers claim that age does not diminish the ability to learn. When alert (and unsedated), most people are capable of extraordinary creativity. Here is a recent finding:

> In general, with good physical and mental health, adequate educational levels and intellectual stimulation, it appears there is not the decline in intellectual abilities with age, as was previously thought. Some abilities, in fact, increase such as judgment, accuracy and general knowledge.*

For older people, then, this is good news. Armed with these findings, they are beginning to fulfill a dream: they are returning to school and resuming their education. Today, in the classroom, what is the latest vogue? White hair, gray hair, a face full of the wisdom-wrinkles of living! Take those two farmers, for example, septuagenarians Pennington and Jones—their pictures are taken for the newspaper as they receive their high-school diplomas. Something to crow about!

"But all this is fine," you protest, "fine and dandy for the community-based retiree. But what has it to do with nursing homes filled with the brain-damaged, the lame, halt and the blind? Surely, for *them* you're not plugging life-long learning, and all that!"

Let us consider the implications of "all that" for the institutionalized. Could it be an idea whose time has come? We have not even come close to recognizing the potential which all too often lies there dormant and unexplored.

First, remember that only a very small percentage of

*Robert Butler, M.D., and Myra Lewis, *Aging and Mental Health* (C.V. Mosby & Co., 1977).

nursing home residents are suffering from *organic* brain damage—some estimates put it as low as 5%. Others suffer from "pseudo-senility" much of which is reversible. Then, there are countless residents—estimated between 25 and 50%—who are relatively healthy in body and mind, but who have moved to a home voluntarily, or for some other important reason. Their communities do not provide adequate or sufficient services to keep them at home—services such as a visiting nurse, home-health care, handyman, companion, grocery delivery, meals-on-wheels, transportation or, most importantly, day care centers for the elderly. And so, with these hundreds of thousands now in residence and thronging to U.S. nursing homes, what about *their* intellectual needs? Well, we know that if a muscle becomes flabby from lack of use, the same is true of the unflexed mind.

Next, count your residents who *could* attend a class or

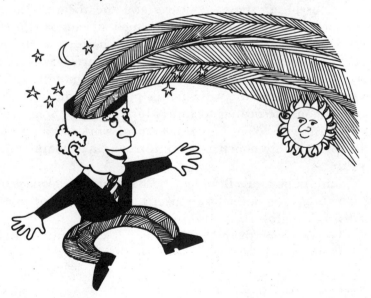

who themselves might be able to conduct one, give a book report, or teach a skill. Did not each one have an interest or expertise? Perhaps one might even play the violin; another might organize a scrap-book, or read Dickens aloud, holding a group of children spellbound. Find out, too, if your local schools or colleges offer tuition-free off-campus classes. Could they come to *your* nursing home? If not, *prod* them. Remind them of that classic life-long learning addict, Oliver Wendell Holmes. When he was asked: "At the age of ninety-two, why are you taking up the study of Greek?" he promptly replied, "Why my good Sir, it's now or never!"

For many years, now, the Soviet Union has promoted the concept of life-long learning. Let us take a look inside a large nursing home, located in Klimovsk, which boasts a library of over eight thousand books. The home provides lectures, poetry-reading sessions, folk-instrument groups, excursions to art shows, concerts and the theatre. In the workshop, residents learn to make such articles as slippers and eye-glass cases; in the garden they help grow flowers and vegetables. For all their work, they earn wages. Each receives a physical examination every three months and is expected to attend the calisthenics program which is mild or strenuous, according to individual abilities. Some residents run every day. This program of work-learning-play therapy is highly beneficial in improving and maintaining health.*

Said Judge Louis Brandeis: "What America needs is not to do things for our fellow-citizens, but to keep open the paths which allow them to do for themselves."

To keep open the paths? This is the wave of the future. Full steam ahead. We must recognize the potential, the vast

*Journal of Gerontological Nursing, October, 1978.

inner resources of our older people, no matter where they reside. Scientific findings which say that *I.Q. scores do not necessarily decline with age* are indisputable. In fact, as Dr. John Valusek, Wichita psychologist, bluntly states: "It is immoral to interfere with the potential of others."

"And now, friend, you *still* look puzzled. Is there something else you want to ask?"

"Yes. What's that eighty-year-old aphasic man saying to those residents?"

"Why that's Mr. Shore. He's giving a book report about the moon landings. And, bless his speech therapist, he's expressing himself very well!"

"And tell me (I'll promise to ask no more), what on earth is that bright-eyed old woman with the fine memory doing over there, looking so well—her joy of living sticking out all over?"

"Why that's Mrs. Ilga Lebedeva. She's one hundred and three!"

P.S. All names in *this* chapter are real. Any similarity to living persons is most certainly intended.

"There are those who give joy—
And that joy is their reward."
     Kahlil Gibran

10 Touch—or The Power Of Your Hand

The Director of Nursing Services was interviewing prospects for the position of staff nurse. Making rounds with them, she observed how each applicant related to the residents. Although all seemed knowledgeable and committed to geriatric nursing, the Director made a quick decision. She chose Meg.

"Why Meg over the others?" we wondered.

Because Meg *touched*. Here, the gentle pat on a shoulder; there the enfolding of a wrinkled hand between her own two hands. Meg understood the power of touch to establish communication and trust.

Mary, one of our nursing assistants, also possessed the gift of touch. She was there the day tragedy struck Mrs. Klein, whose son, David, was dead in a car crash. Wild, unremitting sobs choked the woman, wracking her frail body with convulsions. Nothing that we said or did could ease her anguish. And then Mary took over. With agile fingers, she unpinned and let flow Mrs. Klein's long hair. Circular, gentle strokes of the scalp soon eased the breathing. Closing her eyes, Mrs. Klein fell into a deep, comforted sleep. We lifted her into bed. Mary remained with her a little longer as she resumed the stroking of forehead and temples with an upward motion. Then, at intervals during the rest of the day, she returned to the room—just to be near, to hold her hand, to provide loving support.

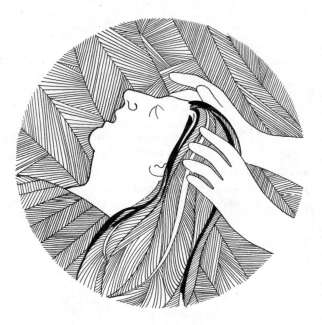

Touch? What is this magic power too seldom applied in geriatric care? Is it not the very bridge to human relationships? Particularly when an older person suffers impairment of sight, hearing or speech? What then remains? Touch — the one sense which, throughout a lifetime, can stay intact. Small wonder that many aging persons reach out to grasp your garment. Just for nearness, just to know you care. Through touch, then, you respond, giving comfort and joy. And that joy is your reward.

To touch and be touched — surely touch is a significant link to self-esteem. Remember, not too many years ago in India, the poor and ill people known as the "untouchables"? Can we comprehend the emotional impact on an outcast who knows he is considered untouchable? Here at home, the very thought puts us on guard. By underestimating the value of touch, do we unwittingly contribute to low self-esteem, anxiety or depression in our patients? How can we let them know they are touchable?

First, revive that ancient and honorable art, the one often relegated to our bottom rung of priorities, the backrub. Yes, the backrub — that perfect sedative with no side-effects which says: "You are somebody; you are touchable!" Include it in your evening care plan; reinstate this ritual so that each resident looks forward to the personal attention it promises. A dab of fragrant lotion, a dab of love smoothed on and watch him slide off to slumberland, at peace with the world. Oh, the power of your hand!

Next, the footrub. Have you, yourself, ever experienced the sheer ecstasy of a foot and leg massage?

"Oh, but wait!" you cry. "Let's not go overboard! I see what you're driving at. No way! Not me. Not on those awful corns, bunions, hammertoes — those — you name it!"

Since you are a thinking (as well as a caring) nurse or

nursing assistant, take a moment now to consider the history
—that's right, the *history* of those feet. From your grand- or
great-grandmother, you have heard tales or seen photos of
the shoes which years ago were considered high fashion—
those pointed, dainty little disasters which wrought havoc
with healthy young feet. Fitted in sizes far too small for comfort, think how they flattened the phalanges, mashed the
metatarsals! And yet, those brave feet carried on in rearing
families, working in farms and factories—yes, in pioneering
the United States of America. You recall the saying: "How
beautiful are the feet of them that serve!"

Most of your residents, then, deserve and will delight in
the gentle kneading, manipulating, massaging—the touch of
your hands which, in many subtle ways, sends the message:
"I care."

Do *you*, like Meg and Mary, possess the gift of touch? Of
course you do—you have only to claim it. Make the most of
it, Nurse, for, as the proverb instructs:

> Withhold not the good from them
> To whom it is due,
> When it is in the power of thine hand to do it.

*" . to have and to hold, a comfort
in sorrow—a companion in joy."*

11 To Have and to Hold

"I take thee to be my (wife) (husband) to have and to hold
from this day forward, for better or worse, for richer for
poorer, in sickness and in health, to love and to cherish,
until death us do part."

It was their fiftieth wedding anniversary. In a little cere-
mony in the nursing home, Ralph and Amy repeated their
marriage vows, reliving that happy day so long ago. Golden
daffodils, yellow roses and candles adorned the lace-covered
table. And now, Ralph was cutting the yellow-frosted cake—
a gift, baked with love, from the nursing home. From the
record-player floated the soft strains of "O Promise Me."

Amy was teary-eyed. Ralph, too, was visibly overcome by the flow of loving attention from staff, family and friends. Even Mr. Case, the administrator, was there, pleased to take part in the celebration as he cordially shook every hand.

And then it was all over. The guests departed. Again, all was quiet. Ralph put his arms around his wife and kissed her. Then Nurse Nora wheeled him back to his room. With a little assistance, Amy walked back to her room where her bedridden roommate, Mrs. Dobbins, waited to hear all about it.

"To have and to hold"?—"'til death us do part"? That night as she lay in bed, the phrases kept ringing in Amy's head. And there were other words which kept resounding in Ralph's mind—"Those whom God hath joined together . . ."

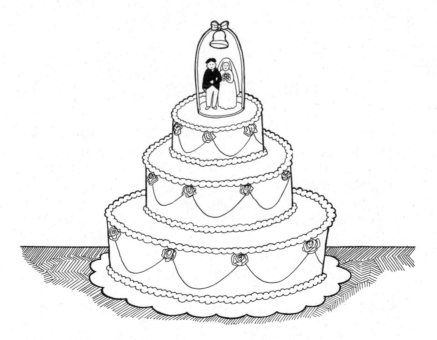

He sighed. "Why may not Amy and I stay together? Nights as well as days?" he wondered.

All of their married life, in sickness and in health, Ralph and Amy had shared a room and shared a bed. But now, in the still of the night, there was no way to lie beside her nor to put his arms around her—tonight of all nights—to remind her again what a beautiful life-partner she was and always had been. Never again would they feel the closeness and warmth of one another nor, with a soft embrace, express their need, their love—never again to have and to hold.

Must they live out their ebbing lives in separation? There remained so little time. But here in an institution, who would understand? Who could know what they meant to one another or what feelings they concealed in their hearts?

That evening, as Mr. Case was driving home, he also relived the joyous occasion. And he, too, turned over in his mind certain phrases—perhaps recalling his own marriage vows—"In sickness and in health" . . . "A comfort in sorrow, a companion in joy" . . . "Let no one put asunder."

On the following afternoon, Nurse Nora wheeled Ralph, as usual, to visit his wife in her room. But today, something was different. The bed next to Amy's was vacant. Photos, clothes—everything—had been removed from that area. Mrs. Dobbins had consented to move in with another friend.

"That bed—it's for *you*!" smiled Nurse Nora. "Mr. Case thought you might like this new arrangement . . ."

. . . from this day forward!

Doesn't it depend on you,
the staff,
to make the

12 Aftermath of Stroke—a Triumph?

Such excitement! Today, Mrs. Park goes home! Her nursing home days are over.

Felled one year ago by a devastating cerebro-vascular accident, paralyzed and aphasic, it seemed that she was beyond hope. But now, because somebody cared, she has made a miraculous comeback.

With tears of gratitude, Mrs. Park slips a note into the pocket of her nurse, Ruth. Borrowing from a favorite poem, she had written:

Bless you, Ruth, for what you have made of me.

Bless you, for passing over all the foolish things
    in me
And for drawing out what no one else
Had looked quite far enough to find.
Bless you, Ruth, for making out of my life
Not a reproach, but a song!

My nurse, Ruth, is a jewel. How can I forget her?
Never discouraged by my dismal prognosis, she went
ahead, gently exercising my limbs and helping me to
form words. An aura of quiet authority surrounded
her. When she said, "Mrs. Park, you will walk again,"
I believed her and was motivated to work for this
goal. That incredible nurse! She opened up doors to
me that had seemed forever closed. To her, the word
"chronic" did not mean "hopeless"—it was her trum-
pet call to arms. Her question was not *whether* to strike
back at stroke, but *how* to convince others that, even
with me, it could be done.
One day in the corridor, I overheard the head nurse
saying: "Ruth, I don't share your optimism for Mrs.
Park. You know what Dr. Morton said."
Complete silence, and then, "Why do you bother,
Ruth? At her age, it's not worth it!"
My heart turned a somersault. But when Ruth returned, her expression restored my hopes. Evidently
I *was* worth it.
To Ruth, I was worth taking the time to help me dress
in my own lovely nightgown—not as simple for her as
to put me in that slit-back monstrosity that makes
you feel like an inmate. Make-up, too, and a pretty
hair-style. One day she exclaimed: "Oh, Mrs. Park,

you look so glamorous you should be a pin-up queen!"
I just about burst.

To her I was worth taking the time, as well, for more
difficult, long-range goals—even retraining for blad-
der control.* Because Ruth recognized my inner
needs, I was able to accept with good grace the rigors
and pains of rehabilitation.

As my improvement became evident, the other members of the staff pitched in, talking as if it were *their*
doing. Finally, Dr. Morton ordered a complete therapy regime—physical, speech, occupational, and rec-
reational therapy—the whole works! Now, everyone
believes in me! I *will* be, I *am*, getting better.

As Jim, my husband, escorts me out of the nursing
home, I'm grinning like a Cheshire cat. They're all
waving good-by. In the excitement, as I hug Ruth,
my cane is knocked over. Words stick in my throat.
Someday I'll tell her what it meant to have a nurse
who looked behind the illness to the real me. Never
pushing, yet always dangling that star before me. Oh,
how I treasure her manner, her way of looking at me,
her touch, the tone of her voice! Always, I could sense
her loving concern.

Our little Chevy rounds the bend on Maple Street.

---

*In the elderly, urinary incontinence is treatable, the success depend-
ing on the cause, the degree of patient cooperation, and the persistence
and devotion of the staff. Treatment involves systematic exercise of the
pelvic musculature, relaxing the detrusor muscle by medication, or surgi-
cal repair. However, when the cause is psychological, it takes only a sup-
portive, understanding staff willing to undertake this task, the success of
which is so important to the self-esteem and dignity of the patient.

There's our house! Oh, and here comes old "Java-Jowls," our St. Bernard! He's lumbering over the lawn to greet his master. Suddenly he spies *me*! Letting out a colossal howl, his great body shudders with excitement.

Neighbors gather around. For a moment I am overwhelmed—transported into an unreal world. But Jim steadies my arm. Now I know I am really home.

Aftermath of stroke—surely a triumph for Mrs. Park and for all who worked with her. But what of other patients whose same, valiant struggle holds no promise for a normal life; no hope for return to hearth and home? What of those

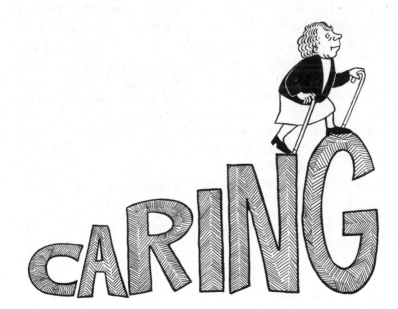

imprisoned in the silent shell of the body, unable to speak or to move? For them, can life hold any joy, any meaning? For a long time, our staff pondered this difficult question. But gradually, through one patient in particular, Mr. Harris, we began to believe it could.

Mr. Harris, severely paralyzed and aphasic, is one of our Hillside patients. He will not be going home. But at times we feel sure that he experiences a measure of inner joy, and when he does, it is perhaps felt more deeply now than before his illness. We wouldn't know this except that through his eloquent eyes, he tells us. We have seen in them a special glow when we speak *to* him, rather than about him, in his presence; when we hear what he cannot say in words. At times we sense in him an inner peace when he grasps the message of hope, conveyed by his speech therapist. Clearly, too, we "hear" his gratitude when we give a soothing back-rub, or gently reposition him. His eyes speak, too, of renewed self-esteem when we meticulously shave and groom him and, with a refreshing rinse, cleanse his mouth and lips. Or who among us doubts that when we hold a rose beneath his nostrils, his expression is one of sheer ecstasy?

Yes, it took a long time, but now we are sure—there is meaning to such a life, as there must be for every life. We came to think of and to know Mr. Harris as an individual, to love him as a member of our Hillside family. And only when this happened could we see the meaning to his life—not only to him but to us. We learned that it matters not one whit what a human being does, earns, or owns. We learned that, in the eternal scheme of things, it matters only *who* he is.

We think that, all along, Mr. Harris has known who he is. For through him, we know better who we are.

Since there's joy
in preventive *geriatrics,*

13 Let's Rethink the Bedsore

"What caused her death?"

"Well, your mother was old," replied the doctor. "She also sustained multiple infected bedsores."

Turning to me, my friend cried out: "But seventy-six isn't all *that* old! Why, oh why, in this era of science and research, are bedsores allowed to develop?"

In her grief, she spoke with perception. For the fact stands: *There is no excuse for any bedsore on any patient at any time.* It is painful. It is preventable. And—although this may sound harsh—it indicates poor medical/nursing care or outright neglect.

The latest available H.E.W. statistics show that in 1975, there were 26,037 decubitus ulcers in *skilled* nursing homes, with the comment that "this is not bad, considering . . ." One wonders, then, if standards are that relaxed in skilled homes, how many exist in intermediate facilities, or in hospitals; how much suffering, cost, and wasted time is involved throughout the United States?

Having worked in many nursing homes in numerous states (as I followed my mobile husband around), I have found the decubitus ulcer often taken for granted in the elderly. Had it not been for one nursing home where prevention was a matter of top priority, I might have joined the True Believers who claim that bedsores are inevitable.

Decubiti, I now assert, are far from inevitable. They are entirely preventable. That certain nursing home, with its share of bed- and chair-ridden patients, clearly demonstrated this. Perhaps a sign over the nursing station made its point: "Success is achieved and maintained by those who try and keep on trying."

"The innocuous term 'bedsore' is dangerously misleading," warns Dr. George B. McDonald, in the *Journal of Rehabilitation.* "The morbidity and mortality associated with decubiti are seldom fully appreciated." Most of us know that they prolong the need for intensive care and delay rehabilitation, but are we aware that, in the doctor's words, "they also produce serious protein and electrolyte loss; chronic infection of the blood (septicemia), bone (osteomyelitis), and tissue (secondary amyloidosis); and even more dangerous diseases such as malignancy and suppurative arthritis leading to joint destruction"?

Nurses know that poor nutrition and illnesses that interfere with blood circulation make a person highly susceptible to decubiti. Special vigilance, too, is required for the patient with paralysis, the comatose, the postoperative and the highly sedated patient, too sluggish to move around. Even depression can lessen a person's will to reposition him- or herself.

Armed with this knowledge, then, our job is clear-cut. We must emphasize prevention . . . *prevention*, that magic word too little heard in America, where "health-care" means "illness-care." Americans do not enter hospitals, nor do they crowd clinics, to prevent trauma. And yet in China and in many European countries, people visit doctors regularly to sidetrack trouble. Part of the problem with decubiti may be inadequate emphasis on prevention. Perhaps some nursing homes should carry the motto: "Bedsores permitted. Here we care, but not enough to give our very best."

Why, then, was prevention 100% possible in that one nursing home? The answer is vigilance. So conscientious was the staff that they would miss a meal rather than skip or

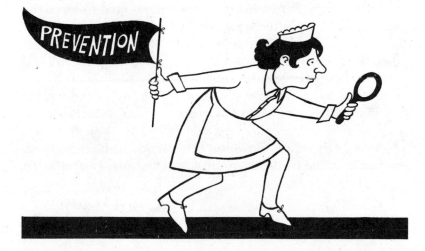

delay the patients' repositioning schedule. No nurse or aide wished to be personally responsible for contributing to a debilitating condition. If a faint red spot on the skin was detected, the staff redoubled its efforts. As members of a winning team, nurses and aides took pride in the fact that their patients were comfortable and that they themselves were doing a good nursing job. And the administrator lost no chance to make sure that the public was aware of the skill and concern that was shown.

Every nurse learns that with prolonged pressure on any part of the skin, a full-fledged bedsore will develop, and that tissues squeezed against anything hard—beds, chairs, casts—even lumps in the sheet—invite clogging of the capillaries and collapsing of the blood vessels. She has seen that ugly hole in the flesh, sometimes larger than a ping-pong ball—the raw bone showing, the surrounding skin swollen and inflamed. But here, bypassing discussion of treatment, we would stress the value of *shared* care. When a resident understands the nursing procedures, when he has some control over what is happening to him, he is encouraged towards the goal of self-care. In the book *About Bedsores*, it is suggested that some patients are able to watch the clock and signal when it is time of repositioning; to use a hand-mirror to keep track of their progress; or, themselves, to find ways of prevention by reducing pressure under a bony prominence.*

Here we simply hope to respark your determination towards prevention, knowing that it can be, and is being, practiced. Open fire, nurse, on this dreaded affliction. Join the battle of the bedsore—rethink the bedsore—rethink the

*Marian Miller, R.N., and Marvin L. Sachs, M.D., *About Bedsores: What You Need to Know to Help Prevent and Treat Them* (Philadelphia: J. B. Lippincott Company, 1975).

crucial part that you play in your all-out goal of stopping it before it starts.

Come to think of it, prevention is a funny thing. *Practice* it and nobody knows the difference—whether it is prevention of bedsores, prevention of constipation,* or whatever. But *fail* to practice it, and there you are, bogged down with extra bed changes, enemas, extra baths, extra sunlamp treatments, extra dressing applications, not to mention all those extra miles of walking down the corridors. Then you find yourself sighing, "Who says there is joy in geriatric care?"

*Write for reprints of the excellent article by Carol Wichita, R.N., "Preventing Constipation in Nursing Home Residents," published in the December, 1977, issue of *Journal of Continuing Education in Nursing*, 6900 Grove Road, Thorofare, N.J. 08086.

14 "Walk, B.I.D., with Assistance"

Doctor's order reads: "Walk." (Not straggle, dawdle, poke along, but *walk.*) And he means it. After all, Mrs. Jones suffers edema, constipation, and insomnia. Physical activity will step up her circulation.

But how often, how well, do we fulfill this order? Either the resident sits—and she sits (her heart muscle becoming flabbier and flabbier), or else—

—watch this hidden-camera movie, filmed as you, Nurse, carry out that "Walk with assistance" order. Ready? Lights out. There you go, entering Mrs. Jones' room.

"Mrs. Jones, want to walk?"
"*Must* I?"

"I'm afraid so," you reply, bored. "Doctor's orders.
"O.K. Help me out of bed."
(You help her so well that she doesn't have to lift a
finger. The walk begins.)
"Come, lean on me. Hold tight!"
(Ninety seconds and three steps later) "Nurse, I've
had enough."
"O.K., Mrs. Jones. That's plenty of exercise for one
day. Here—sit down."
"Thanks, Nurse. But next time, let's not go so far. I
am tired."
(Still clocking, the camera follows you to the nurses'
station, where you chart: "Pt. walked, as per doctor's
order.")

Now, that order didn't specify *what kind* of walking, did
it—how much, how long, how far? That's up to you. But the
kind you settle for is just about perfect for promoting physical and mental stagnation. Assuring continued reliance on
laxatives and "sleepers," it also perpetuates feelings of de-
spondency.

"But I walked her—followed orders," you say. "What
can you expect at her age?"

Plenty, Nurse, plenty. You expect too little, allowing
premature deterioration before your very eyes. Inactivity
and forced dependency are undermining her health, her
self-image. When Dr. Paul Dudley White, heart specialist,
championed the use of regular, mild exercise for a well-
functioning circulatory system, he meant the old as well as
the young.

Indeed, even when we withhold enthusiasm from the
care we give, we are expecting too little. So Mrs. Jones is

depressed? She's slow? Why fall prey to *her* moods? You're the one to set the tone.

Last summer, in Oregon, I clocked a slug as he moved up a window-pane (he's the most inert, slow-moving creature around); he covered a half-inch in forty-five minutes. That about equals the pace you set for Mrs. Jones when you walked her!

Now let us move ahead three months in time and see the result of Mrs. Jones' so-called "exercise program." Most of this time, Mrs. Jones has been resting. She has been "walked" occasionally, yes, but *who* gets the exercise? The nurse, not she. Deeper depression has set in. Her feet are always cold. Immobility aggravates the constipation. Tremors have developed. All interest in life drained, she has lost resistance to infection. Hospitalized for pneumonia, there she gets some more "much-needed rest." Three days later, she gets the best rest there is. She's "resting in peace."

The doctor had ordered *walks*, remember? B.I.D. walks? But you never quite took that seriously. After all, you figured, this is a *"rest* home."

I'm for scrapping that phrase "rest home." Why not make this an "up-and-at-'em" home? When the doctor orders walks, walk the resident. March him! Work up to longer, faster body movements before it's too late. Strengthen him, build him up. Soon he'll put that slug to shame—break his speed limit. Make that heart muscle beat strong—*stronger*, for each day a patient stands still, the treadmill pulls him a step backward.

With all your enthusiasm, motivate him—get him to believe in his rehabilitation, to believe in himself. For whatever his *dis*abilities, his *abilities* far outnumber them. Spruce up that circulation. Walk him as though *you mean it*. And before long he will be saying: "Up and at 'em" and will walk, B.I.D., *without* assistance, as though *he* means it!

*Many residents find in their religion the ultimate dimension of joy.
As part of total care, then, should a nurse, or a nursing assistant try to
meet their spiritual needs?*

15 O Be Joyful in the Lord!

"Who *me*? Provide *spiritual* care? Why that's the job of the
chaplain!" exclaimed Becky, the young nurse. "I don't even
know what you mean by 'spiritual needs'! I wouldn't know
where to start. Besides, haven't I enough to do on my shift?"

It is true, every word. Especially when the nurse herself is not an active churchgoer. How then can she recognize,
let alone fulfill, a resident's spiritual needs?

Before you tune out entirely, Becky, let us observe Mrs.
Randall, a resident in your nursing home. Although, with
others, she attends the nondenominational Sunday or Sab-
bath service in the lounge, this resident misses the religious

life to which she had been committed. Back home she had also attended church on Holy Days, had arranged altar flowers, fasted, tithed and reserved quiet time for Bible study. But here she cannot depend on those rituals to provide a sense of belonging, a close relationship with her God. She longs for the outward and visible signs of her faith.

Gradually, an ache wells up inside her. She begins to feel like driftwood, tossing aimlessly on a vast sea. "Oh!" she cries out to the nurse. "The void in my heart! Why, oh why, has God forsaken me?"

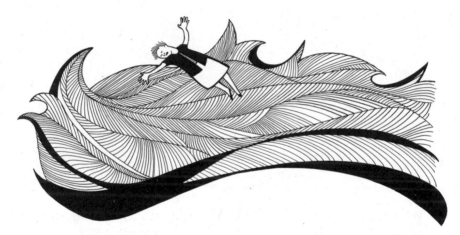

If at this moment Becky makes no response, Mrs. Randall may withdraw. But what can Becky say? Indeed, *should* a nurse intercede in such a clear call for spiritual counsel?

"That's the job of the clergy," she insists.

Yes, it is. But not every chaplain feels at ease in a nursing home. Some may not have come to terms with old age itself, nor with its reminder of their own mortality. Further, how can a religious leader, of whatever faith, reach out at all times, when needed, to each parishioner on the list? There

are too few shepherds to tend the sheep. Have you not observed the chaplain who hastily enters a patient's cubicle,
rushes a ritual, then vanishes? They do their best but, spread
too thin, can rarely spend more than a moment with any
one resident.

These days we talk of "total care." Mind and body. But
often we forget that it is mind, body *and* spirit which com-
prise the total person. And since you, Nurse, are in direct
contact each day with the resident, it is *you*, primarily, who
hold the key to observing and assessing his or her deeper
needs, *you* who can help provide solid support the moment it
is needed. (Ideally, you do so *before* a crisis arises.) And so,
confronted with Mrs. Randall's spiritual S.O.S., how do you
respond? She wants to know why her God has forsaken her.
You have a choice.

1) Ignore that cry of anguish? Change the subject, slough
her off with a lame "Don't worry, God loves you." But
wouldn't this turn her feelings inward to fester even more?
Never again may she feel free to share them with you, nor,
perhaps, with any other nurse.

2) Even though the pressure of other duties hangs heavy,
can you affirm her need, sit down with her, listen caringly?
For you know that these few moments, in the long run, may
require less time and energy than dealing with a full-blown
crisis, should the chaplain not be immediately available.

3) Far more effective, however, is a nursing interven-
tion which you, or any staff member may apply. Be venture-
some! Give this one a chance. You say you have forgotten
how to pray? Then, of course, you are not about to pray out
loud. Still, there *is* one thing you are accustomed to doing,
that is, caring. And you *are* used to caring out loud. And so,
when a resident reaches out for spiritual solace (or even
when he doesn't, but your sensitive "antenna" picks it up),

there is one beautiful step you can take—one that is as simple as asking your Mrs. Randall if she wants a drink of water. Ask if she would like you to pray with her.

"But in such a situation, I would feel uneasy," you say. That is understandable. But just let the heart take over. Post a DO NOT DISTURB sign on the door, take her hand, bow your head, and observe a moment of silence. She herself may be the first to voice her supplication. Or, if by now you feel at ease, just speak her need in a few sincere words, such as:

> Lord, Mrs. Randall is feeling so alone tonight. She feels that her family and we nurses are too busy to visit very often. She feels so far away from You. But You are with her every step of the way. You are with her now, easing the pain, calming the fears in her heart. Tonight, let her sense that You are close. Give her a restful sleep in the knowledge that You care, that we *all* care, and that we love her. Amen.

Then, squeeze her hand or gently put your reassuring arms around her. And tonight, because you have affirmed her spiritual need and shared this joy, Mrs. Randall will sleep more peacefully.

When a resident feels heavy-laden, expressing alienation from God and things of the spirit, is there any medication, any treatment more powerful than prayer?

In time, Becky, you will feel comfortable in giving this kind of care, may even want to share your thoughts with other staff members, even to the point of charting: "Pray with Mrs. Randall PRN." And you will have established "continuity-of-prayer" as well as something tremendous— "in-home spiritual care" for those who, like an unwatered plant, may be close to withering.

In a survey, although a majority of nurses said they would feel comfortable praying or Bible-reading with their patients, at least half stated they had never done so. And, as Sharon Fish and Judith Allen Shelly say in their book *Spiritual Care*,* there is need for serious in-service training on how to recognize and fulfill to a greater degree the spiritual needs of many patients. Certainly, the geriatric patient.

Total care. The integration of mind, body, and spirit. And of the three, spiritual care may well become your most rewarding responsibility. For, as we blend faith with our nursing duties, we experience joy within ourselves—the same joy that we give away.

Finally, Nurse Becky, here is your greatest blessing. You discover that you *are* adequate! You *are* as qualified as anyone! You *can* help your nursing home residents, once again, to feel the loving presence of their God.

And now, "be joyful in the Lord," as both of you

". . . walk eager still for what Life holds
Although it seems the hard road will not end—
One never knows the beauty around the bend!"**

---

*InterVarsity Press. Downers Grove, Illinois 60515, 1978.
**Anna Blake Mesquida.

And finally,
our ultimate satisfaction
and joy is

16 To Make Meaningful Their Days

Your geriatric resident—who is he (she)?

Same as we. An American, a child of God, a human being moving ever closer to the "top of a mountain high."

But with one difference. He's a step ahead. As Pearl Buck so well expressed it, he's one who has "come a little farther in the experience of life." He's had more time to serve his country, his community, his next-of-kin.

Renewing our commitment to him, we offer this dedication:

> "Mine eyes have seen," but eyes are slow to understand. Now, at last, our hearts have seen. You are

beautiful. You are a proud people.

Even when we trampled your hearts and dignity, your love kept shining through. Your trust never faltered.

And now, as your shadows lengthen, and your evening comes, we light a candle—symbol of our desire to lighten your darkness and show you that we care.

For brightly it shines to warm you with our love, to make meaningful your days, and, at the last, to surround you with a soft glow. For truly—*you are America's grand generation!*

"To make meaningful your days," we've promised. Is not this our greatest challenge? Easier said . . .? Not when the nurse stretches, full length, her imagination. Not when we latch on to life roles. As the staff did with my father.

"Good Heavens, Father," I fussed, "today it's beans on your vest. Last time I came, it was egg on your chin. *I'm* hauling you out of here! I'm finding you a nursing home where you'll get more meticulous care!"

"Oh, no!" cried my 88-year-old dad, almost plunging from his wheelchair. "I won't hear of it! Who would counsel the lonely? Who would assist at chapel services?"

Father had been a minister, accustomed to leadership. Here he could live out his life role. He was still "somebody." Weighing the choices, I conceded. Thereafter, I simply scraped off the beans and egg and praised the Lord that there was continuity to his life—there was meaning to his days. For six more years, Father remained highly motivated until, joyfully, he kept that date to meet his Maker.

In another nursing home, can staff awareness of life roles help "ornery" Mrs. Ross?

Oh, how it jangles their nerves—her habit of sneaking

off the premises! Former director of a ceramics business, she heads straight for her old shop, where, of course, she gets the red carpet. There, she's part-time Queen-for-a-Day.

Upon her return, however—you guessed it—scoldings. A few "naughty-naughty's," and she's right back in her role of Mrs. Nobody. As a substitute satisfaction, what if she were to be appointed Assistant Activities Director in charge of Ceramics?

Or, in the lounge, doesn't that lonesome piano long for some elderly virtuoso to give it the "Tea for Two" treatment? Encouraged to practice, just watch the venerable Mr. Higgins (ex-piano teacher) burst his buttons as friends exclaim: "Didn't know *you* could play!"

Each of those residents had a life role. Old Mrs. Bates— wasn't she a wonderful grandmother, known for her scrumptious sticky-buns? And Mr. Stein over there—I hear he was a crack carpenter by trade. How can this information be tied in with their present existence?

So your patients are clean, and you're kind to them? That's enough? That's all they need? Hold it! Hear that commotion up there? It's Dad, pounding his cane on Heaven's floor. "Hey, you nurses down there," he's calling, "that's not the half of it!"

Creative geriatric nursing means more than pills, pulses, and prostheses. It means that we know who the resident was, who he is, and who he can be. It means that we lighten his darkness, show him we care.

Keep the candle glowing. Make meaningful their days, that, as they move upward, they may smile and say:

> Age is the top of a mountain high,
> Clearer the air, and blue.

A long, hard climb, a bit of fatigue,
But oh—
What a wonderful view!

[*Author unknown*]

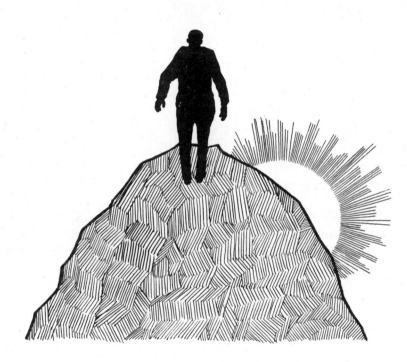

*We strive to bring joy
into the lives of our residents.
And now, at the end
of her journey,
we support Augusta
as she experiences*

17 A Good Death

Death is not just the surrender of life,
but a positive act worth doing well—
an act people need help to accomplish.*

Surely each one of us wants a good, painless, peaceful, and dignified death in familiar surroundings and in the presence of those we love. This ideal is described by the Greek words *eu*, meaning good, and *thanatos*, death.

But what is a good death? Let me tell you about one that will occur within the next few hours.

*Arthur Gordon, *A Touch of Wonder* (Old Tappan, N.J.: Fleming Revell Company, 1976).

Friday Afternoon, 2:00 P.M.

Here in her home, death is claiming my 82-year-old Augusta. I was called in on my day off to "special" her. And a very special and dear and personal friend she is. I'm now holding her hand, speaking quiet words of reassurance.

For three years Augusta has been in and out of the hospital. She has suffered many strokes. Now, a "final" CVA brings on more paralysis and helplessness. I rush to make the emergency call. I stop short. Why? Must she again be subjected to tubes, needles, suction machines—all those scientific marvels that she so dreads? There in an institutional atmosphere our Augusta would again be "distributed" among the staff—everybody's, yet nobody's, patient because of the impersonal system under which medical care is generally administered to the terminally ill.

I ask her sister: "Do you want her to re-enter the hospital?"

"No," she quickly responds. "Here Augusta knows the touch of your hand, the sound of your voice, the one-to-one relationship that has meant security."

Relieved, I see the decision is made. We will keep her at home for the remainder of her time.

It is not easy to watch Augusta's temperature spike to 104 degrees, nor to see the precipitous drop in her blood pressure. Moistening her lips and repositioning her, I stand by as she slides into an exhausted sleep. Now I recall the time that she so earnestly said to me: "Nancy, in case of crisis, let me stay home."

4:00 P.M.

Augusta is now awakening. Her skin is hot, but she is

calm. It is good that she has emotional support in her final human experience. I wipe her brow. She gently presses my hand, telling me what her aphasic sounds could never convey — that she is all right, content and under no strain, even in the knowledge that she is dying. Her dignity and her humanness are preserved. Fortressed by a devoted sister and by being at home where she knows affection, she is being spared perhaps weeks or months of the unnecessary anguish that might have resulted from the artificial lengthening of her life.

4:35 P.M.

And now, Augusta, your breathing is becoming irregular. Your heart is tired, making its last effort. It would be unkind if I were now to feel your pulse or flaunt before you a cold stethoscope. Instead, I am putting my arm around your shoulder, holding you secure and helping you to cross the threshold. It won't be long now.

5:00 P.M.

Augusta, your lips and mouth are again becoming dry. It is not too late to swab them gently one more time. Do I discern an almost imperceptible smile, as if you were trying to tell me this helps a little bit?

5:10 P.M.

Your minutes are numbered, Augusta. It is because of you, dear, that I feel compelled to write on this subject. I bid you farewell, knowing that you have been helped to embark on your journey. Yours will be a calm passage. Those of us you leave behind are grateful that you are experiencing a "good death." Your years of anguish are soon to be replaced by release and repose. As I watch you lie there, your soft white hair draped over the pillow, I see that you are at peace, for you know you are not alone. You have your faith. You have your God. I will keep my vigil until the very end.

5:11 P.M.

And now, Augusta, I see the last vestige of color draining from your cheeks. You have only a minute or so more. Yet I can only reflect, this is a good death; this is a perfect death. Sharing this experience with you gives me an awareness of the deeper meaning of life in its closing hours.

5:12 P.M.

Your time is here, Augusta. You breathe heavily. A deep sigh. You take your final breath. Your heart stops.

It is over.

Rest in peace, our beloved Augusta. Your light perpetual will shine—will always shine, here in your home.

In remembrance of Augusta, and for all who labor to nurse the ill and aging, we ask:

> Lord, support us all the day long, until our shadows lengthen and our evening comes, our busy world is hushed, the fever of life is over, and our work is done. Then in Thy mercy grant us a safe lodging, and a holy rest, and peace at the last. *Amen.*

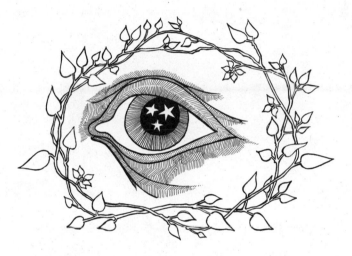